# Are You An Intelligent Massage Therapist?

## Then You Need To Be Massaging At A Luxury Day Spa

## By Heather Leigh

# Are You An Intelligent Massage Therapist?
## Then You Need To Be Massaging At A Luxury Day Spa

Heather Leigh lives in San Diego, California with her two sons, cat muses, and Australian Shepherd. She is the author of *Hey Little Baby*, a perfect baby shower gift, *Scout and Ellie,* a funny middle grade chapter book about a boy and the elephant living in his backyard, and *Red Nectar,* a young adult novel about Emily, a teen with the talent of telepathy in a world that kills for her skill.  Her books are available through her blog listed below:

www.heatherleighauthor.blogspot.com

Published by Heather Leigh


Leigh, Heather, 1968-

Are You An Intelligent Massage Therapist? / Heather Leigh

# Table of Contents

Chapter One:
How Do You Break Into This Highly Sought After Job?

Chapter Two:
What Are The Three Resume Tips That Will Get You An Interview?

Chapter Three:
What Needs To Be Known About Spa Before The Interview?

Chapter Four:
What Are The Five Things To Know About The Interview?

Chapter Five:
What Do You Need You Know Before Your First Day Of Work?

Chapter Six:
Don't Be Afraid Of That First Day — Be Ready

Chapter Seven:
What You Must Do and Not Do During Intake Interview

Chapter Eight:
How To Give The Best Massage With The Least Effort

Chapter Nine:
How Do You Get Your Client To Rebook

Chapter Ten:
Leaving a Job

# Are You An Intelligent Massage Therapist? Then You Need To Be Massaging At A Luxury Day Spa

## By Heather Leigh

Busting into the day spa massage therapist field was one of the best career moves I have ever accomplished. Everyday, I was surrounded by a plush, luxurious work environment in which my clients were always happy to see me. As most were there to relax and feel good, the attention they asked for leaned toward medium-pressure massage — nothing that would hurt my body over time. . The spa does the advertising, buys and cleans the linens, and provides the clientele. In order to attract clients, a high-end spa will promote health, beauty and tranquility. What better environment is there for you to work in?

I loved my job, made great money, had an awesome network of friends to hang out with and trade massages, and was able to constantly be making people feel better. I loved that decade of spa work.

Why luxury spas over other places to work? As much as we joined the ranks of natural health practitioners to help people, we still have bills to pay. Plus, if you are working at a place that is heavy in clientele needing deep-tissue and focused pain relief, the faster our own bodies can be worn down. Day spas that allow you to keep your physical health will make it easier to stay in the field and help more people. And the more expensive the spa, the better the tips will be.

Having worked for chiropractors and physical therapists, I can say that while that work was rewarding in being able to assist others in becoming pain-free, it was hard on my body. Chain spas that I served time in gave me extra money for Christmas, but the pay was low and the constant flow of needy people wore me out—I felt like I was working in a human body fix-it factory. Throughout my ten years I always held onto my own small out-call clientele business, but the driving and set-up time never fully compensated for the pay I received. For two years, I rented a room for my own business. While I enjoyed getting close to the regular clients and watching their health improve through my hands over time, I still had to market my business, wash the linens, do the scheduling, and buy the product. It wore me out.

The years that I spent bringing people relief in a chaotic world, and helping many to rid themselves of pain were wonderful. I am honored that I was physically and emotionally able to serve so many people. The spa harmony that clients and I were able to be a part of enabled both of us to lead more productive, healthy lives, for which I will always be thankful.

According to Associated Bodywork & Massage Professionals, as of February 2013, there were 1,319 massage therapy-training programs in the United States, and 320,000 trained therapists. There are many graduates out there wanting jobs. This book is here to stand beside you, leg bolster and eye pillow in hand, and bust down the spa door and massage your way into an awesome career. Let's get going so you can work and relax.

# How Do You Break Into This Highly Sought After Job?
## Chapter One

The fact that spas are so wonderful to work at means the desire to get hired is great. Massage schools are pumping out certifications daily and the graduate population is growing — it's a popular field.

There are three main reasons why the competition to get into this tight market is intense:

1. The therapists often know one another and stay in their good paying positions for years. This gives little vacancy for the new kid on the block.

2. Being a newbie to spa work, it is not expected that you will give a great massage.

3. Spas want you to have prior experience.

Don't despair — see these as challenges to overcome and not mountains that block your way. Let's go through them together.

**They Are A Tight Net Bunch**

The first issue of being unknown is to get known. Do you have any friends, acquaintances, and friends of friends in the industry? Make your desire to work in a spa known to them. Ask if they know of any place that is hiring.

<u>Network</u>

Networking is a breeze nowadays with computers. Post on every social media outlet you subscribe to that you are looking for spa work, as long as this information is only going out to friends and family.

I once needed a Chemistry tutor for my son and after posting my request on Face Book, a friend of a friend of a friend recommended someone. The tutor was in our living room two hours later getting my son ready for an exam. The friend who originally got my posting lived eight hours away!

You never know what spa is searching for a therapist and people love to help. Be sure to get the name of whoever gave the information. Ask that person if you can let the management know they sent you. If it all works out, he or she will get credit for filling the position and you may have a new friend in the business. Also, give a massage to the person who gave the referral; this is valuable information and they should be rewarded.

<u>Book All Over Town</u>

Another trick is to book a massage at the spas you want to work at. When you receive your massage, ask your therapist if that spa is hiring or if they know of another place. Therapists tend to be friendly — they wouldn't last long in the industry if they weren't. Be sure to ask if they know of any place that is hiring on-call, seasonal, poolside, or event staff. These are great ways to get your foot in the door.

If you are a student, you may balk at the thought of paying for a massage at a high-end spa. The rates are often higher than your daily paycheck. But almost every spa has specials and discounts. Group-on, local magazines and the spa's website may reveal something that won't bust your wallet.

When I had completed enough training that I could be hired by a spa, I booked massages at every spa in town. Yes, it was more than I could afford, but I did it any way. One of the places had a reputation at my massage school as being a terrible place to work. As a result, no one applied there — except me. When I went for my massage, I decided to be open to what I observed and not what I had heard. What I discovered was that the staff was friendly, and the spa pretty, clean, and had a comfortable-well decorated lounge that offered fruit and cucumber water. My therapist was wonderful: friendly, personable, and gave a relaxing, awesome massage. At the end of the treatment, I asked her about open positions and learned there was an extra room that the owner had been trying to fill with another therapist. I turned in my resume the next day and was hired two weeks later.

The owner was strict and on the aggressive side, and my co-workers were professional gossipers. The up side was that the tips and pay were great, the boss turned out to be honest, thoughtful, and fair, and the gossiping co-workers were like a tight-knit dysfunctional family that knew how to have fun.

If I had listened to my classmates put down that spa and not gone to experience it for myself, I would never have found a job that turned into a great place to work for over two years.

Yes, I was lucky to find a spa that negative rumors kept my competition light, but no matter how few therapists applied there, I would not have been hired if I were not able to give a great massage.

## Newbies Can't Massage—Bash That Myth!

The next obstacle to overcome is in making your massage feel like your hands have been relaxing people for many years.  This is done through:

- Practice, practice and more practice

- Being confident

- Knowing what people are looking for

- Being knowledgeable

<u>Practice, Trade, and Give</u>

The more you're practicing massage, the better your massage will be. Don't undervalue the benefit of giving out free or extremely cheap massages — learning how to massage is a hands-on experience (I couldn't resist the play on words!). Trade with your classmates. As they have had the same training, you will gain insight as to how your massage may feel and what you think you could improve upon. Give free massages to friends and relatives. You will quickly become a popular person to be around!

Teacher Experience

Also, be sure to book with your teacher for every different type of massage learned. They often give student discounts. Going directly to the source, you will experience how that type of massage should feel.

## Be Confident

Often, I can tell a beginning therapist by the feel of their hands in the first touch. There can be an almost unperceivable shaking, a nervous energy, and a lack of confidence that is palpable. Know that however little training you have received, most people seek massage because they want to be touched. I don't mean this in a sexual way, but with a spirit of love and acceptance. This is a stress-filled, anxious society we live in, and being touched in a healthy, safe environment can be like discovering a secret garden in the middle of a chaotic city.

## Peanut Butter Difference

Also, every therapist has something different to offer. A co-worker once told me of a massage she received that was the best she had ever had. Afterward, she fretted that she would never be that good.  But then, she thought, massages are like peanut butter; there is creamy, chunky, natural, mass-produced, and everything in between.  There are so many types available because people have different tastes.  While one person may not be transported to a peaceful existence by your touch, the next ten may just love it.

Feedback

Be sure to get feedback from every client. Ask in a way that doesn't sound like you are trying to bolster your self-esteem, or make it about you. Ask if:

- there was anything that they would like to experience more or less of in the next massage
- you covered everything they needed done
- they are relaxed

Most people will just say the massage was great and give no real suggestions or advice. If it is a friend, press for honest criticism. Be ready and okay with being told that there are some aspects that you could improve on. It's better to hear this from a friend than to have a paying customer who won't say anything but won't rebook with you.

Subscribe

Be sure to subscribe to a massage magazine. My favorite was the one that came with my massage practice insurance. The magazine featured articles about new techniques and equipment, tips and ideas in better serving clients, and helpful products. It was a wonderful source of connection to people who had been in the business for years and were ready to pass on their knowledge.

I've heard it said that a therapist must give one thousand massages before they are any good at the practice. I strongly disagree. I've had massages at schools that were excellent and massages from people in the business for years that were dull and made me want to ask for my money back. If the person getting off your table is healthier, more relaxed, and in a better state than when you started, then you are giving a great massage. Practice and learning more techniques will serve to make you an even better therapist.

**Get Experience**

Prior experience is like the puppy chasing tail syndrome. How can you gain experience if you can't get hired in the first place? This question goes round and round in every career. Luckily, as a therapist you have more options available than most other professions.

## Business Owner

Start by having your own business. This may be easier than it sounds.

Check the local and/or state requirements on when you can start practicing. The school you are, or were, learning from should be able guide you on where to ask. As soon as you legally can, set up a business of out-call clients, meaning you go to their house.

(*An aside tip here: don't go to someone's house who you don't know or wasn't recommended by a friend. Once there, call someone within earshot of the client and let him or her know where you are at and when you will be done. I've never had any safety concerns during out-call visits, but playing the 'better safe than sorry' game is always a good idea.)

Because I lived outside of city limits, I was allowed to legally massage in people's homes after one hundred hours of massage school learning. Where my cousin lived, she was also a therapist, the requirement was three hundred hours. These amounts can be completed in just a few months. So check the requirements before assuming you can't do anything.

There are not a lot of therapists willing to do house calls. The time it takes for set-up, hauling around your table, traffic, gas—everything combined drives many away from the practice. However, it is a great way to get the experience wanted on your resume, practice on bodies, establish a reputation, and help people who might not like or even be able to get into a spa.

For the client, to have someone come to his or her house is awesome. It can be difficult to find a trustworthy person. There are many people who don't like the spa experience, especially men or old-schoolers who think it is a feminine luxury that they want no part of. And if you are responsible, do a good job, show up on time—you will be an invaluable part of many people's lives!

As soon as you have a license to practice, you can make up a name, get business cards, and pass them out to your friends. If you have a friend or family member paying you one dollar for a massage, you are now a professional massage therapist and this can go on your resume. As a professor of mine used to joke, if you are ten miles from your house and have a smidgen more knowledge of something than the people you are talking to, you are an official expert in your field.

Chain Spa

Chain spas are the places that charge a monthly fee to get a massage a month. They are known by their name, are inexpensive, and have many locations. Although the work is often harder and the pay low, it is another way to get your foot in the door of experience. They generally hire people straight out of school. Plus it is something else to put on your resume.

When I needed some extra money for a down payment on a condominium, I spent three months at a well-known chain spa. I've known co-workers who did the same. We had the same attitude that while we preferred our other job, it wasn't a bad thing to have some extra money.

Everyone I worked with at the chain spa was fresh out of school, or still attending. I wish they had read this book because there were so many mistakes I saw therapists doing that lost them money in tips and rebooking--it made me feel like yelling or crying or both. So, thank you for reading this book and taking the time and effort to be a better therapist!

Small Spa

Be aware that many of the luxury spas do not consider chain spa therapists to be ready to work for them. Luxury day spas are a different venue. A small local spa may be another option. Many of the smaller places are looking to have a therapist on-call, or rent out a room. Seems like every hair salon, chiropractor, and nail care spa is advertising that they offer massage. As a result, there is a high demand for therapists.

There are things to consider:

- do they want you to stay at the spa for walk-ins
- will they pay you an hourly wage to wait
- would they be open to you being on-call

- if they want you to rent the room, how many massages would you have to do in a month to pay for the room
- could you rent the room with a co-worker
- do you already have a clientele list
- how many clients could you expect from the spa
- do you have to bring in your own linens and oil

A small business may be just the thing that works for you for the time being, but investigate thoroughly before you start working.

Small local day spas usually look better on a resume than chain spas. Chain spas are known to hire just about anyone with a massage therapist degree. The day spa may be harder to get a job at with no experience, so talk up your own business. Make it sound like you have many clients and have been doing it for a while, with out lying.

Of course, the goal is to move beyond out-call, small spas and chains, and into a luxury spa. During this transition period, be grateful for the experience, resume building, positive reputation you are gaining, and the ability to help others. There is a light at the end of the tunnel called luxury day spa, but the scenery along the way is good, too.

# What Are The Three Resume Tips That Will Get You An Interview?
## Chapter Two

Your resume needs to be professional, show experience, display a history of working in the attitude of a therapist, and make me want to grab the phone and get you in for an interview. It is often seen before you've even met a supervisor at the spa, especially when applying on-line. It needs to be eye catching, informative, grammatically correct and stand out above the stack of other resumes on the bosses' desk. And you have one page to do this in.

1. Pad Your Resume

This means that you want your resume to look like you've been active in the business for years. Here are some tips to get you going:

## Learn as many styles that you can

In massage school, there are all kinds of different massages to learn. To know which ones to take, find out what the spas that you are interested in offer.  The most common are:

- Swedish
- Deep Tissue
- Shiatsu
- Thai
- Reflexology
- Pregnancy

Take these classes as soon as you can, and then branch out into what the spas around you are offering, and what you are interested in — you should be enjoying your career.

Massages that offer other specialties generally teach them to their employees, so you don't have to learn every technique before applying. The six listed should be enough to get you qualified, but knowing more will give you more confidence, enable you to better serve your clients, and make you more employable.

Beyond school, you can also attend workshops, lectures, and economical on-line courses.

<u>On-line Courses For Hands-On Work?</u>

Yes, surprisingly there are many subjects to learn on-line that can be posted on your resume. Before hot stone massage was popular, it was not offered at the school I was attending. I bought a DVD, my own stones and turkey roaster, and found friends willing to lay down and let me learn on their backs. After enough practice, and not having burned anyone, I added stones to my list of resume skills.

Other things I've learned on-line are nutrition recommendations, giving Vichy showers, about ayurveda medicine, and tips on massaging the face. How-to techniques can be found for free on websites and You Tube. There are also on-line companies that will give course information, a test at the end, and a printable diploma. The cost is often very low, and more items to add to your thickening resume.

## Weekend Workshops and Hour Long Courses Count Too

Once you are on one roster for massage therapists, it will seem like course ads follow you like a zombie after fresh meat. I think I received one for myofacsial release at least once a week, if not more.

If that's not enough to satisfy your hunger to learn, I've seen advertisements at libraries, yoga studios and in community college catalogues. There are so many fascinating massage techniques available in different places — it makes the career you've chosen even more enjoyable.

Take whatever courses are within your budget and that you even halfway think you will enjoy. Education is a great gift to give to yourself and the clients who receive the benefits of your growing bag of tools.

Make sure to update your resume with every course you take.

### Work At A Variety of Places

While it does not look good to have had many short-term jobs, it does look good to have volunteered your healing hands at Charity Walks and marathons. Just think how popular you'll be at the end of the Three Day Breast Cancer Walk. I've had friends offer their time at hospices, hospitals and nursing homes.

### On-Call

If you apply at a spa and they tell you they are not hiring, offer to be on-call. Spas will often massage entire wedding parties, and groups of employees being appreciated by their employer. Valentines and Mother's Day is two weeks of busy-ness at all spas. When a spa offers a big special or limited time discount, they often need extra hands to help carry the load. And I used to joke that I paid my mortgage by covering for therapists who called in sick at the last minute.

So while the spa may not be hiring, it does not mean they don't occasionally need an extra therapist. If you can get an on-call position, you can smack that spa onto your resume, gain experience, earn some extra income, and be first in line for when they are ready to hire.

In the previous chapter, we talked about getting work at different spas. Starting from school with whatever jobs you can get will allow you to not only pad your resume, you will be practicing what you are learning while getting paid. I've even had a job offering chair massage poolside for the summer at a resort hotel. The tips were great and we were under a cabana in the sun with a DJ and children laughing in the background. What could be better than that?

## Proudly Post Your Certificates and Affiliations

Some of the courses I've taken outside of school offered certificates to show you had learned the material. When I took reflexology, it was a three-month course and at the end I could show that I was a certified reflexologist. These are great to have in your portfolio.

Any related affiliations you are or have been active in can go in that resume. Are you a member of the ABMP, Associated Bodywork and Massage Professionals? Not only do they offer affordable body worker insurance and an informative monthly magazine, you can claim membership to their society. These affiliations make you look serious about your practice and give professionalism to your resume.

Massage clients often believe that we know about nutrition, alternative medicines, aromatherapy, herbology — anything to do with the body and taking care of it. Taking courses about anything to do with natural health and alternative medicine will benefit you, the client, and that resume.

Another reason why massage is an excellent career; you can become aware of so many things to pass onto your client. Your life will always be stimulating!

## 2. Getting Write Down To It

Resumes should be one page. Supervisors are busy people and want to know about you and what you have to offer quickly. But you also want to stand out from the stack of papers on their desk. This is done by using concise language that clearly states what you've done, how well you did it, and uses the best possible word for each sentence. Every word counts.

Making Every Word Count

Make the descriptions interesting with just the right adjective. You want to sound like you know a lot from each position you have ever held. For example, if you were a sales associate at a clothing store, state that you enthusiastically sold fashionable clothing to high-end clients. For my stint as a food server at a casino, I wrote that I efficiently served food and drinks to promote a quick return for the gaming clientele. In other words, we had to hurry with the food so they could throw more pennies in the slot machines.

<u>Throw Out The Adverbs and Adjectives</u>

A trick I learned in a writing class was to write out what you want to say. Then remove all adverbs and adjectives (adverbs are words like happily, joyfully, enthusiastically; adjectives are the descriptive words like bright, nice, beautiful). What you have left after their removal is your actual story, or here it would be the description of your previous employment. Now, rewrite the sentence, sprinkling in the adverbs and adjectives that are the exact ones that will describe what you did. Did you joyfully serve a client, or did you actively listen to the client to discover the best way to serve them? Which sounds more like what you would want from your therapist?

Add those adverbs and adjectives like salt to the soup; too much and you come out looking like a beginning cook, too little and no one will take a bite.

## Every Job Description Must Slant Toward a Massage Theme

Write your resume to show that you consistently worked in a way that portrays the traits common to our helping field: being a great listener, caring about guest's needs, and a desire to help others. Also, time management skills, self-marketing and retail sales are desirable. Use these and similar words to describe your jobs. Make your resume look like they are about to hire the ideal employee.

You weren't just flipping burgers at a fast food restaurant, you were cooking with efficiency and skill to serve consumers in a timely manner. You never simply stocked shelves, you ensured that supplies were properly placed so that customers could easily find what they needed.

A cook at a fast food restaurant or someone who stocked shelves, do not at face value sound like any thing to do with massage therapy. However, with creative writing, you can sound like the type of person who will continue to serve others in the way of the therapist.

3. Get Help In Every Nook and Cranny

Being an expert in writing resumes is not a requirement to getting hired. Just about everyone working today has written a resume, so that means there are plenty of people who know how to do it. You don't have to reinvent the wheel. There is plenty of information on how to make a wheel and a resume and you can easily access what others have already learned.

Trading Is The Perk Of The Therapist

Trade in your field is one of its greatest benefits. There are few people who will say no to a massage in exchange for help in resume writing. Find a friend who is excellent at writing resumes, get them on your table, then to their desk to assist you in creating an enviable resume. Of course, you should probably work on the resume first — after the massage they will be too relaxed to write anything of value.

Research Resume Formats On-line

In this era of learning via computer, you can know just about anything you want to know in minutes. Look up resume formats, tips, and samples. There are services for hire that will look at what you post them and tell you what it needs to be awesome.

You can also use the computer to send your resume to friends and family for their input and suggestions. You never know what advice a friend could give that will be just what was needed to create perfection.

Pull your history together from every known source in your working world to get your resume thick. Write it in a fashion that makes you look like you were born to be a therapist. Bring in those who have gone before you, and are good at it, to help with making that resume the one that will get you in for an interview. You have the tools, you have the knowledge, now go and create the best resume that shouts to the world that you are ready to massage.

# What Needs To Be Known About Spa Before The Interview?
## Chapter Three

So you were called in for an interview!

Congratulations! If this is a busy day spa, getting that

phone call can be difficult. Now that you've

successfully jumped that hurtle, it's time to do your

homework. Luckily this is simple homework — think

of it as an easy 'A'.

<u>Research</u>

Before you go in, research the spa. If it is large enough, it should have a website to get most of what you need to know. If not, hopefully they at least have a brochure you could pick up a day or two before the interview. Look at their menu to see what they have to offer. You don't have to know how to do every massage they offer, but you should at least know what they are.

One spa I worked at had a Balinese massage. It had been put together by a supervisor from what she had experienced in a trip to Bali. There was no way we could have learned this except through learning it at that spa.

Know the Basics

Even if you have yet to be trained in Thai, hot stone, pregnancy or shiatsu massage, you can know what they are all about. Again, that wonderful resource called the internet can be utilized to download a video clipping of these therapies in action. Or, better yet, do a trade with a therapist who specializes in one of the practices.

Don't worry about not being pregnant to receive a pregnancy massage. When I took that course, I practiced every week on my stepfather. As far as I know, he'll never need that type of massage, but he enjoyed the relaxation and I gained a new skill.

Prenatal Advice

An aside here to promote the learning of pregnancy massage. Many therapists are reluctant to perform this service. Either they are not comfortable around pregnant bodies, or don't feel they have the proper training. For me, this meant that when prenatal was requested at a spa, I was the one who would get booked for it.

In addition, therapists are often booked with pregnant women even if they aren't trained in this unique service. But pregnancy is more than just giving a gentle massage. There are places on the body that need an extra soft touch and areas that need more focus. The woman may ask you a pregnancy related question and you should be able to answer. Also, there are a lot of false rumors and old wives tales out there that still haunt the service. The biggest one is to not touch the feet, when in reality, this is the place where a lot of attention should be given. And, finally, ways to better serve women in this wonderful time of their life is an awesome gift to be able to offer someone.

## What The Heck Is A Vichy?

I've never heard of a school teaching Vichy shower treatments because they don't have the equipment. As each spa does it differently, and learning it is as easy as taking a shower, don't worry about not having performed one. But, back to the web, watch one being done or read about it. Especially if you think this might be something to soothe itchy vichy skin, you better search the web to see what this awesome service is all about.

Look At All Spa Services

Don't limit your research to the section for massage services. There are often add-on services that estheticians or nail technicians do that the therapist may occasionally do also. For instance, one place I worked at did hot wax treatments for the hands and feet. It was advertised under nail services, but was also performed by therapists and estheticians.

If during an interview you are asked if you can perform a particular service, it is fine if you cannot, but you should at least know what it is. If you are asked, let them know that you are open to learning it and if hired will search out ways to learn it.

Body Wraps

Body wraps are often performed by therapists and are not traditionally learned in school. They are easy as wrapping your arm in plastic wrap but take practice to perfect, maintain relaxation, and ensure proper draping. Again, this is another service not generally taught in school, so find a way to see one or receive the service yourself.

Products For Sale

Beyond the services, spas generally sell products. Some are savvy enough to sell the oil, lotion or product that are used in services. If you already know and can talk a bit about what they are selling, you will be way above your competition. All it takes is a few minutes of researching via internet about their product line.

The last spa I worked at sold Pure Fiji which is made by a mother and daughter team from the Fiji Islands. They hire the locals to make the product and use the money made to give to the community. This is the type of information that you can discuss during the interview — congratulating the hiring supervisor on using such an awesome product.

You don't have to know every detail of the products they sell, but at least know what they are using. A few minutes of web time goes a long way in knowing your stuff and feeling confident before meeting your possible future supervisor.

In review the things to know are:

- spa services
- products offered

- fundamental knowledge of thai, hot stone, pregnancy and shiatsu massage
- what a Vichy shower treatment is
- the basics of body wraps

A busy spa that pays and treats its employees well is going to have resumes flying at them constantly and be giving lots of interviews when they go to hire. Having a resume that portrays a professional therapist with the skills needed to serve their clients will give you a huge boost to getting called in for an interview. If, on top of having a strong resume, it is obvious that you have done your homework about them, your chances of getting hired will expand greatly. You will show yourself to be someone who goes after what they want and is willing to learn. Show that you are interested in the spa, and they will show an interest in you.

# What Are The Five Things To Know About The Interview?
## Chapter Four

### 1. Keep Your Attire a Step Above

Wear something that is one step above how the therapists working there are dressed. You want to look like you could start work that instant, and are the best dressed of the bunch. If the uniform is to dress in black, wear black trousers or skirt and a nice shirt. Don't wear long sleeves so they know you don't have scary, offensive tattoos or eczema.

Quick tips:

- no jewelry, except wedding band
- light make-up
- short nails

- absolutely no cologne or perfume — it can mingle with products they are selling or a guest might not agree with your tastes

Look and (don't) smell like a therapist ready to work.

Once when reviewing applicants with my supervisor, we decided not to hire an otherwise very capable therapist because she had bright red lipstick, over-done, thick make-up and loud colorful clothing. Our thinking was that if she wore this to an interview, what would she wear to come to work? She would scare away some of the best paying, conservative guests.

2. Simple Yet Needful Items To Bring

Have on hand:

- extra resume, in case yours was lost

- folder so resume remains presentable

- a pen--may not sound like a big deal, but it makes you look efficient

- appointment book or electronic scheduling devise at hand to book that second interview. You do not want to have to say 'I'll get back to you'

These little touches will help you feel more relaxed because you will be presenting yourself as a professional who knows what they are doing. You won't have to say you don't have something, have to ask to borrow a pen, or be shuffling through your belongings to find something. Be the Boy or Girl Scout ready to fix any request coming at you.

3. Therapist Body Language

The interviewer wants to know how you will be with client. When you meet him or her:

- shake hands firmly

- speak clearly

- be confident

- say their name and thank them for calling you in

These things sound obvious, but I've seen so many fail at these simple niceties that they need to be repeated and thought about before you go in.

When they walk you to their office, look around. Compliment the spa décor or something you find intriguing. Chances are, the supervisor has put some of his or her touches in to the surroundings and they would enjoy hearing that others like what they have done. Honest appreciation is always good to hear and will get you started on a good footing.

During the interview, look at the supervisor like you would a best friend telling you the story of meeting a new exciting guy or gal.

- sit up straight

- don't fidget

- listen carefully to questions

- repeat a rephrased version of question

- think before you answer

Picture yourself as the interviewer. What would you want to see from the person sitting across from you? What body language demonstrates a person eager and ready to work in their spa? Who would you want to work with on a busy day, face Monday mornings with, and trust with your clients? Be the person that you would hire to make the spa the best place to be in town.

## 4. Boring Questions They Will Ask

There seems to be a book somewhere that tells the interviewer to ask the same questions for every job on the Universe. While this is unimaginative, it saves you from feeling like you are stepping into an unknown dark cave. Here is the list of the most overused questions in the working world:

- Why should we hire you?

- What experience do you have?

- What would you do if a client were disagreeable or complained?

- What is your worst trait?

- Are you comfortable selling products (only used if therapist is expected to sell their stuff)?

Let's break these up to a level you can deal with.

First, they should hire you because you are perfect for the position. Be ready to talk your self up into someone who is a team player, excellent at servicing guest's needs, taking care of the customer, and gives a wonderful massage. What is it about your personality that people are drawn to? Why is your massage so great? Why do people like you? Everyone has traits to admire and this is your moment to let them shine.

Second, previous chapters have suggested ways to gain experience beyond having given your boy/girl friend a great shoulder rub. This is the time to verbalize every skill you have, especially the ones the spa offers. You could also say that you notice there is one that they offer you have not learned yet, but saw a course somewhere to learn it. That will show that you have been doing your homework and are truly interested in that particular spa.

Third, a disagreeable client usually just wants to be heard. Take the time to actively listen to what the client has to say. This means stay focused on what they say, repeat back what you think the answer is, and then offer the best solution that you can. Often, this will diffuse the situation. If they are complaining about you, don't argue or try to defend yourself — that just makes you look guilty and confrontational. Instead, remain calm and treat the complaint as a suggestion from which you can learn. If the guest is angry, let it be their anger. Keep your emotions separate and your professionalism at the forefront.

Now, take in what I have written and put that into your own words. Mix it with your ideas. As long as you sound like you have a legitimate plan on how to deal with difficult guests, this question won't be a stumbling block. That's a good thing to have ready for an interview, and for when it actually happens in a workspace.

Fourth, turn your worst habit into a good trait. For example, I would say that I get so caught up in wanting to learn something, that I don't quit until I have the knowledge. You might be so into being organized, that you go overboard about having shelves stocked properly. A therapist may be so into helping their clients that they have to always be aware of the time, as they know that ending on time is crucial to a smoothly functioning spa.

If you can't think of a bad habit that you possess, I'm sure an ex-boy/girl friend could help you out. Whatever your trait is, figure out a way to make it sound desirable — but don't be obvious, keep it subtle.

Fifth, of course you are comfortable selling products. As you have already researched what the spa is offering, you can tell the interviewer something positive about the lotions, oils and body scrubs on the front shelves. You can say because the products are so great/healthy/good for the skin/locally-made, it would be a pleasure to offer them to guests. You don't need to be a high-pressure salesperson to be a therapist, just one who is comfortable giving product information and suggestions on which to purchase.

5. Questions For You To Ask

At the end of the interview, it is often asked if you have any questions. Be ready to answer with something like:

- Is there an opportunity for me to sell the products that you use?

- Do the massage therapists or estheticians do the body treatments (such as Vichy showers and body wraps)?

- If there is a massage unique to the spa, ask what it entails?

- If the spa looks busy, are they planning on expanding?

- What type of clientele usually visits them?

- ask questions that show you want to work at that particular spa

Do not ask about pay, tips, scheduling, or commissions — these are second interview questions. Asking too soon makes you sound greedy. You will want this information before you accept a job from them, but at this point you want to portray a person who is thinking more about the spa and the client than monetary gain.

If you don't feel like too much of a geek in doing this, practice being in an interview with a friend. You'll feel more confident if you've already said what you will be saying again later.

Give It A Week

If it has been a week since you have heard from the spa manager, give him or her a call. Say something like, "Hi! I just wanted to check with you on the status of the hiring process and to let you know I am still interested."

A spa supervisor is extremely busy. The therapist who calls back when they have a stack of resumes and notes to review, is much more likely to get the job. It shows that you still want the job, they won't have to find your number later, and that you are motivated. That one call could get you hired.

If they have already filled the position, let them know that you are interested in being an on-call therapist. This is a great way to get your foot in the door. Many therapists don't show up for work at the last minute. I used to joke that I paid my mortgage covering for therapists who called in sick because they had a hang over. One called in and said the stars were misaligned and she wouldn't be able to work that day. They are notoriously flaky for a reason. Or the spa may book a group and need extra therapists for just a few hours.

I especially liked being on-call for one or more spas in addition to the main one I worked for. That way, if my number one job was slow that day, or it was my day off, I could answer yes if an on-call place asked me to come in and work. Unexpected money is always a good thing!

<u>Second Interview — Yey!!!</u>

A second interview is only given when they are serious about hiring you. Give yourself a shoulder rub in congratulations!

It is the time that you will be giving the manager a massage to show you have what it takes to 'wow' their clients. They are standard because they need to know first-hand what the client will be receiving. Here are some tips:

- review the section on meeting the manager
- ask what you need to bring, such as your own lotion or music.
- act as though you were working on a real client--even if the supervisor says, 'just do what you normally do,' tell them that you normally ask what the client wants
- make the supervisor feel like they are getting the real thing. Understand that this person has a busy, stressful job and could probably use a massage more than any guest who walks through the front door
- read the chapter on giving a massage

- pretend the manager is a VIP client.

After receiving your ultra relaxing massage, the manager will hopefully ask if you have any questions about working there.  Now is the time to bring up pay, tips, scheduling, and commissions. The questions to ask are the same or similar to the ones asked if you get a position at a small local spa:

- do they want you to stay at the spa for walk-ins

- will they pay you an hourly wage to wait

- does seniority effect scheduling and how

- is pay based on hours worked and/or commission

- is gratuity included for guests in their bill

To Stay Or Not To Stay

Some places want you to stay there so that walk-in clients can be readily seen. I've done this for no pay and at places that pay minimum wage while you wait. Others will put you on-call during your assigned time and let you leave when you are done working, provided you keep a cell phone on you and can return within a pre-set time limit. All ways have their advantages and disadvantages. At a busy spa, being there ready for walk-ins often works for you and the spa. But if business is slow, there is no hourly wage, and you are not supposed to leave, you may feel that your time is being wasted.

Booking Ways

Research how the booking is done. There are two main ways to book between therapists: Seniority, and how many hours therapists work during the week. Most places go with Seniority; they book the therapist who has been there the longest the first massage, and then go down the line until they get to the therapist who was most recently hired.

I worked for one place that filled the entire day of the most senior therapist before going on to next therapist. The newest therapist had to wait until everyone else was fully booked before getting a single massage. If the spa is constantly busy, this can be okay. But generally it is not.

Even though I was one of the longest employed, I objected to the practice. Everyone needs money. I didn't like being busy while others were sitting around making nothing. It just wasn't fair. Luckily, the next manager stopped this practice.

### Gratuity Included

The best incomes are often generated at spas that include the gratuity in the bill. Although most people tip the standard twenty percent, clients from different countries, those new to the spa scene, and guests with Gift Certificates often don't know they are supposed to tip. Doing an expensive, three hour Ritual that takes up half of your shift and then not receiving a tip can really hurt your paycheck. And of course, the more a massage costs, the higher your tip will be.

Whatever the supervisor says in answer to your questions, don't give a reaction when they tell you. Nod your head, smile slightly, and say hmm when they tell you something you disagree with — like a friend explaining why they are getting back together with the jerk they just broke-up with. Decide if how they are managing things will work for you after the interview. If you are at the stage of just trying get in, take what you can get. Again, some money is more than none and experience is essential.

If you are extraordinarily lucky and are hired before you leave — it can happen — ask to schedule a time to come in so you can review procedures before that first day. The next chapter tells what you will need to know.

When you leave, again shake hands and do all the niceties given to an honored guest. Tell them thank you for their time and that you hope to hear from them soon.

I hope you leave with a smile on your face and an expectation to be hired soon.

# What Do You Need You Know Before Your First Day Of Work?
## Chapter Five

Woo Hoo! So you landed your first spa massage job! Huge Double Congratulations!

When you receive the great news, schedule a time to come in to review their procedures and to know where products and linens are kept. Even if the supervisor says they will show you the day you start to work, ask politely if you can come in before that. Tell them you will feel more comfortable on your first day if you already know your surroundings.

Another therapist can show you around in fifteen minutes. Most therapists are friendly and want to help. Also, it helps them to have a co-worker who knows what they are doing—not have to show them around when they are busy. I have seen so many new therapists come into work and because it was a busy day, never get trained in spa procedures. It makes for a tricky, confusing first day.

Know where to find these things:

- towels, linens and oils—in room and extras
- ritual and treatment supplies
- list of scheduled clients and their treatments (usually on a computer)
- water for client

- pick-up and drop-off area for client (Relaxation Lounge)

- dirty linen baskets

- extra blankets and pillows

- pregnancy pillow or what they use

- employee area for breaks

- massage room clock (they're often put away between massages)

- eye pillow

- foot bolster

- kleenex for crying guest — it happens

- stones for massage and how to heat properly

Other good things to know:

- what you are responsible for cleaning

- time you have between clients

- can you change the music and temperature of room

- how to adjust the massage table

- if you are expected to sell products, ask about the procedure

- how to know which room you will use for each treatment

- how will you know if schedule changes during a massage

That last thing to know is important. The schedule of clients you will be seeing rarely stays the same throughout the day. While you are in a room massaging, the spa receptionist may book you with a massage for as soon as you are done with your present one. Or, scheduling can change to accommodate a walk-in. You need to consult the schedule between every massage, even if you think you already know what you are supposed to do. Busy spas are constantly changing and you are expected to keep on top of your shift.

Knowing these simple things will make your first day at least a teensy bit less scary. You may still have butterflies in your stomach, but at least there will be a few less.

Don't Be Afraid Of That First Day — Be Ready
Chapter Six

Are you ready for that first day? Do you have on your uniform, clean, pressed and ready for success?  Get in to your new work place early with a smile on your face; ready to meet co-workers and help people to relax.

After you've put your stuff away and checked your schedule, you'll be getting your room ready for that day's list of clients.  Doing a bit of preparation before a guest comes in will help keep you on time and calm.

The Three Things To Ease Into A Great Massage Are:

1.  Have Room Ready

Just like any good hostess waiting for the guests to arrive for a dinner party, you want to have a clean, inviting space.  Be ready for your client:

- Keep your room clean and free of clutter. *Client wants to relax, not feel like they need to clean before you start*

- Know where extra blankets, towels and pillows are kept. *Women with big breasts may need a rolled hand towel placed at an angle between breast and front of shoulder. People who have recently gone through some sort of surgery may want to lie on their side for comfort.  Clients with lower back pain often like to lay face down with a folded towel placed under hips and lower abdomen. Be ready to make suggestions and have the*

*towels, pillows or blankets ready to help them*

*be as comfortable as possible.*

- Know what to do if you discover client is
  pregnant. *Many spas will not treat during*
  *first trimester, or require a doctor's note.*
  *Does spa use a pregnancy pillow? Know*
  *where it is kept. Many people think that*
  *massage is not any different for pregnancy*
  *and are surprised to discover that it is very*
  *different.*

- Double-sheet. *Most spas give short time*
  *periods between massages to clean and*
  *prepare for next person. A common trick is to*
  *have several sets of sheets already on the table.*
  *Then when you go back to the room with only*

*a few minutes to get ready, you can whip off*

*the used sheets and have new ones already in*

*place and ready to go.*

- Have oil, eye pillow, and bolster ready

  but out of sight.

- Give extra beauty for more costly

  treatments. *If you are doing a more*

  *expensive, specialized treatment, then have*

  *your room look extra beautiful; let them know*

  *it is worth the money they spent. I would*

  *often gather a few flowers to put around the*

  *oils or room for ritual treatments. Make them*

  *feel special for having chosen this more*

  *expensive treatment*

- Lower lights and have relaxing music going. *Client should be entering a place of relaxation and comfort.*

- Hide the clock in a place that you can easily access once they are on table with their eyes closed. *You need to be able to end on time, but client should feel like they are in a place in which time does not exist and everything is being taken care of for them.*

2. Meeting the Client

Be ready to make a great first impression with every client. Think of yourself as a host welcoming a potential wealthy business client into your home. You wouldn't shout, 'hey, come on in,' through the front door when you heard the doorbell ring. You would go to the door and welcome them into your home. This is how you want the client to feel, like a welcomed guest that is honoring your home with their presence.

Most spas have a relaxation lounge where you pick up clients. They differ on whether to call client by first or last name. First is better as last names can be difficult to pronounce correctly. If the policy is to say last name and your guest has a challenging one, say it the best you can and then ask how to say it correctly. Let them know that even the pronunciation of their name is important to you.

Let them know you care right away. Tell them your name and shake their hand firmly. People want to know the therapist is ready to give a firm massage if needed. Look client in eye and speak clearly. Be friendly and happy to meet them. This all sounds like basic common sense, but I have seen many therapists treat clients like a friend coming over to hang out, or a body to get money from. Show you care and are capable from the first moment.

When you leave the relaxation lounge, offer to carry any water, book, or anything they may be carrying. Treat them like royalty.

I don't recommend offering water, as then they may need to use the restroom during massage. If client is pregnant, ask if they need restroom before massage — pregnant bladders are small.

3.  The Walk To Your Room Is A Chance To Connect

As you are walking to room, talk about how great the spa is. Tell about other treatments that are offered, what spa has that is unique, and décor that you appreciate. Let client know this is the place to be — not in those words but in implication. People want to go where others think it is the greatest place to be.  We tend to believe that what is popular must be better.

Also, ask about client about himself or herself. Where are they from? Are they locals? Are they in town for business or to meet family? You might mention that you like their blouse or shoes, something honest that you will both feel good about hearing. Keep any conversation light and easy-going. That way, they will feel more comfortable with you. They are about to let you massage their naked body and will probably feel better knowing you are not some crazy kook.

Do not ask about what they want in massage, or what is going on with their body, or any ailment on the way to your room. This is all confidential stuff that should not be discussed in a hallway.

Do not talk about yourself or complain. This time is for the client; it is their time for relaxation, pain and stress relief — not to hear about someone else.

This person you are about to do body work on is paying you well, trusting you with their bodies, and coming to you for help. Let them know from the moment you meet them that they made the right decision in coming to this spa and allowing you to help them. It is an honor to be allowed to help people on such an intimate level. Make sure they know you feel this way through your actions and kindness.

# What You Must Do and Not Do During Intake Interview
## Chapter Seven

Your client is now in your room at this fabulous dream job. What do you do now? They are expecting you to know what you are doing — to be the professional one. Well, if you're not feeling it, fake it 'til you make it.

If you are holding your self like a pro, standing up straight, remaining calm and relaxed, listening to what they have to say with the care of a therapist, then you will portray a therapist. First because you are one, and second because you will look like what they were expecting.

Ten Things To Know To Easily Be The Pro:

1. Open Door For Clothing

When you are in the room with client, stand near the open door. Many people will start undressing if you close door. I've never felt comfortable talking with a naked person standing in front of me while I am standing there fully dressed. It's weird.

2. Talk About Treatment

Start out by telling them what treatment they have scheduled and give a brief description of it. Incorrectly booked treatments do occur. The spa receptionist may not understand what they have booked client with. They often make appointments for treatments they have never experienced so don't know how to describe them properly. Brochures with the descriptions are often unclear and inaccurate. You want to be sure client is getting what they want.

3. Upgrades

The most common upgrade is from a Swedish massage to a Therapeutic massage. This is because many order a Swedish, not knowing the difference between that and something that is more site-specific or uses more pressure.

Swedish massage, or Relaxation massage, is about relaxing. It utilizes long, effluent strokes with light to medium pressure along the whole body. When a client talks about treating specific areas, or deep tissue, they probably need to upgrade to a different massage, often called a Therapeutic massage.

Know your spa's policy on the difference. Some spas, the client pays the same price whether the pressure is light or deep. Most places charge extra for site-specific deep work. Now is the time to have everything clear on what they will be receiving--not during the massage when they trying to relax.

An aside note here: while it may not seem like a big deal to go ahead and give a more expensive Therapeutic massage without saying anything to the client, it can hurt you later. When clients come in with a friend, they'll usually talk about their experiences. If one discovers that their friend got more pressure for free—you don't want to be a part of that complaint. Or, the client who got the free therapeutic upgrade may comeback and expect the same from another therapist. This seemingly nice gesture you gave to a client can snowball into something big later on.

When you discover that they really need the upgrade, politely ask if they would like to spend the extra money on a Therapeutic massage. Save yourself future grief through open communication.

Other upgrades may include aromatherapy, special oils, or an extra half-hour for a foot rub. Knowing what your spa has to offer can bring you a higher commission. Be sure to let the front desk know what you have done — you want to get paid for your efforts.

4. Intake Sheet

Some places require Intake sheets that have a picture of a client and a place for ailments to be written about, usually chiropractic offices and chain spas. Massage schools teach students to use them so new therapists often think they are needed. If you really like them, then go for it. To me, they seemed sterile and over-kill. Especially in a day spa that has a high client turnover rate, storing a sheet about every client can get crazy. And people are not stagnant in what is troubling them. The arm you worked on last week may feel fine now but the left leg may be causing pain.

If you work in a place with a lot of regulars, I recommend keeping your own box of 3 X 5 inch cards with basic information about the clients you see on a regular basis. These can easily accessed and don't take up much space. Such things as having had back surgery, stay away from knees, likes light massage on arms but extra deep on shoulders. Also, personal information like where they work or how many kids they have. It is nice to know this stuff when they come back for massage and it is hard to remember the lives of every client.

5. Medical Conditions

Ask if there are any medical conditions or rashes that you should know about. Usually it's that they have muscle tension in their shoulders, an area they hurt doing sports, or that they have ticklish feet. If they do say something serious, don't show alarm. Talk with them about the best treatment to help within the time limit. If the client has a condition that you think will be worsened by massage, such as severe varicose veins, state how you feel. Stopping a massage is rare as massage is helpful for just about everything. However, if you feel strongly about something, be polite yet firm and end your time together.

Now is when it may come out that they are pregnant. Don't be alarmed, just be ready and know what to do or say. If you are not qualified to treat pregnant women, don't be afraid to cancel massage. It is better to end it now than to put a pregnancy at risk. There are many therapists who think it does not matter and will just give a light massage, but being trained in pregnancy massage is a big deal. I used to teach pregnancy massage and there are things that can be done that could potentially harm a baby during a massage. I also recommend that you get trained in pregnancy massage. Don't lose clients because you didn't take a much needed class.

Clients are often embarrassed by a rash they may have and not say anything. But with the lights dimmed, to suddenly find a rash you can barely see is not cool.

If they tell you they are under going cancer treatment, ask if they are receiving chemotherapy. If they are, I recommend that you stop the massage. Chemotherapy drugs can go through their skin and onto your hands, harming you. But especially important is that massage can speed up and intensify the effects of the drugs, making massage unsafe for your client. Tell them that while you really want to help them at this difficult time, massage is not good for them right now.

6. What's Going On?

Ask, "What is going on with your body"?

Listen and repeat back a summarized version of what they have told you, without sounding like a parrot, and tell them what you think they want done.

For example, they might say, "My feet are ticklish, go light on my lower back and I hold my stress in my shoulders."

You can answer with something like, "I will go over your lower back and give extra attention to your shoulders with more pressure. Should I try to relax your feet or not touch them at all?"

Sometimes there can be work you can do before massage starts, like wrist work from tui na, or acupressure to treat a headache. This impresses people when you can do this and makes them feel like you really care and know your stuff.

This is probably the most important time to really be aware and remember what you have heard. I believe the most common reason that people do not return to a therapist is because what they asked for was not given. When they tell you that their arm biceps hurt from playing too much tennis and you barely go over these muscles, chances are you have just lost a rebooking. Listen and remember to give the extra, or less, attention to the areas they tell you. Giving the massage they want will bring re-bookings and a happier client.

7. First Timer?

If you haven't already, ask if they have ever had a massage before. First timers will need more instructions and guidance. A massage addict will go through these procedures quickly.

8. Pressure

I used to ask what kind of pressure people want before touching them, until someone said to me, "how do I know what kind of pressure I want until I feel what kind of pressure you give?"

This made sense to me so I quit asking. After that, I started everybody with a medium pressure and then asked after about five minutes into the massage whether they want more or less pressure from me.

My pre-massage question about pressure preference changed to, "During the massage, let me know if you want more or less pressure, or anything different from me."

With this statement the client knows it is up to them to let you know what they want. Also, they are aware that you are open to doing things differently.

9. Site Specific Pain

When a client says they are experiencing site specific pain, have them point and touch the area. Saying their hip hurts could mean anything from the top of the iliac crest to the attachment point of the hip flexors. And most people think that the rotator cuff is one muscle, they don't know that it is a group of muscles. Touch lightly where they are showing you so you know for certain where to focus.

9. Review

Before you leave room, very quickly review what you will be doing. You want this whole intake process to be personable and friendly, efficient and timely. Don't spend too much time cutting into their massage time. Although some clients will spend so much time trying to tell you about every ache, pain, and injury they have experienced, that they talk away the time needed to help them. Try to politely let people know you only need to know what is relevant for the massage right now because you want the time to be able to work on them.

10. Questions From Client

Ask if they have any questions for you. Especially for first timers, the most common question is if they should take off their underwear. Unless you are not comfortable with this, or it is against spa policy for some weird reason, the answer is yes. However, most first timers are not ready for complete nudity. Tell them that while most people take off their underwear, it is up to them if they do, it is their comfort zone that is most important.

Tell client where to place clothing, or robe, and shoes. They will be naked in a darkened room. The last thing they should have to worry about is where to hang a robe.

Suggest that they take off necklaces and big loop earrings so that you can work on their neck. Also, have them remove their watch so that you don't get oil on it. Bracelets and rings are easy to work around. Especially have them keep their wedding ring on. You do not want something expensive to be lost in your room. Show them where to place their jewelry on the counter. Ask that they do not place these things in their robe pocket as they can fall out easily or be forgotten. After you have searched through a huge pile of dirty robes and linens to find jewelry that a guest has lost, you will always remember this procedure—I've learned that lesson more than once!

Ask them to lie face up or down, depending on your preference, with their head on the table or in the face cradle. Make it clear what you want them to do.

Tell them to lie *between* the sheets, so you don't walk back into the room with someone lying on the table face up with nothing covering them: awkward moment.

Make sure that you fold back the top sheet when explaining all of this to them, so that they are clear where to get in. If you have double sheeted, and they pull back several sheets, every sheet they pulled back will have to be washed — uggh!

Let them know you will be back when they are ready so they know they have a few minutes. You want them to feel relaxed about getting into the table, not having to worry that you will be rushing back in a moment later. Come back within a few minutes to begin massage. I've seen many therapists go and make a phone call, or hang out with co-workers. This is not okay on so many levels that it seems pointless to lecture on why leaving a client for a long time is bad, so I will assume you would never do this.

Talking with a client about what will be happening during their time is like writing a clear outline for a story. If it is all set up before you begin, you both know what to expect. You can go through the massage knowing that they will be receiving what they want and they will feel more at ease. A few minutes of review gives for a more relaxed environment.

# How To Give The Best Massage With The Least Effort
## Chapter Eight

Now starts the peaceful time between you and your client. Everything has been set up to give the massage perfectly tailored to their needs. Keep the atmosphere calm, quiet, and peaceful. The client is counting on you to give a much needed hour of respite from a busy world.

<u>Stepping In</u>

When you step quietly back into the massage room, be appreciative that this person who does not know you has just allowed himself or herself to be naked and vulnerable around you. They are probably face down and cannot see you; talking briefly and quietly will let them know that it is you, not some random stranger who was walking down the hall.

Ask if:

- the music is to their liking

- it is at volume that they like

- they are comfortable

- they want a bolster under their legs

Only ask about the temperature if you have a way to change it, such as turning up the air conditioner or draping on a blanket.

What To Do With Chatting

Talk briefly and quietly. This is their time to relax. If they are chatty, answer their questions while allowing for space for them to quiet down. Many people new to massage may be nervous and will cover their nervousness with chatter. Allow for a few moments of talk and then invite them to listen to the sound of their breathing, feel their body heavy and melting on the table. Most people will take this hint and quiet themselves. If they continue talking, give soft, quiet answers. Do not talk about yourself. Again, this is their time, not yours.

The only time I am open to talking is if the client is someone who gets regular massages. Then they already know about being quiet and have made the choice to talk. If you are in a spa, be aware that there may be people in the next room disturbed by noises coming from your room.

The Great Massage Story

Massages are like a story; there is a beginning, middle and ending.

1. In The Beginning

The beginning should be an overall relaxation of the entire body. From massage school, you should know techniques that quiet the entire body, such as light compressions or gentle rocking of each limb and the back done above the sheet. Allowing the whole body to know relaxation now, will create a body more open to receiving deeper work during the session. As a good friend and esthetician once told me, "if you can get a client to completely relax, you will have a life time customer."

If you like to massage the scalp, now is the time to do it—before applying oil to your hands. Be sure to ask client if it is okay to massage their scalp. Some people may be going back to work and don't want their hair messed up—or simply not like scalp work. If they don't want oil in their hair, place a hand towel over their head, assuming they are face down in a face cradle, to prevent the oil from spreading. I was so accustomed to continuing effleurage strokes up the back and through the hair that the towel served as a reminder not to do this.

2. Middle

This is the bulk of your time spent with your client. The type of massage, and what you've agreed to give extra attention to, will be given during this time.

## Order

Which order of the body area to be worked on is up to you. Most therapists start first with the back and then continue on to the arms and legs. After a scalp massage, I preferred the feet and legs first, and then back so that they would be the most relaxed to accept work on those stressed out shoulders. Try different sequences to find out what works best for you.

In a busy spa, because ending on time is so important, it is best if you stick to the same sequence when possible. Make sure you have practiced getting your timing perfected before working in spa so you don't end up spending forty minutes on the back and have no time left to get to their arms.

The back is where most clients want the most work done. Generally, expect to spend about fifteen minutes on the back.

## Arm Trick

A trick I learned was to work on the entire arm, front and back, while they are lying face up. This works if you hold the arm out and slightly up, but be sure to keep it supported. It sounds funny, but I would stand like a flamingo with one knee resting on the side of the table and use that leg to support their arm. Practice different techniques before trying it with your paying guest.

## Pressure Check

Within five to ten minutes of the massage, ask quietly if they want more or less pressure from you. If they say it is fine, then great, you don't have to ask again. If they want more or less, change to their instructions. Be sure to ask again a few minutes later.

Even though you can tell a client repeatedly to let you know if they want any changes made, most people are too polite to say anything. But this is their time and bringing them to their highest comfort is your priority.

<u>Their massage</u>

Now, if you remember nothing else in this book, remember this: give the massage that the client wants. Even if you know that their shoulders are a mountain of stress and screaming for deep tissue but they ask for a light massage — give the light massage. If you feel that their top layer of fascia is tight and know that myofascial release would be perfect for them, but they are not open to the idea, do what they want.

Personalize each massage. Just because you give a great massage that 'everyone' loves, doesn't mean that the person you are working with will love the same one the previous client did.

If the client comes back for a second visit, you could say that you noticed that their shoulders were tight and might they be open to try a firmer massage around those tight areas. If so, work somewhere between what they said they want and move toward what you feel will help them more. Don't scare anyone away by not listening to want they want.

When I first started and people told me what they did not like about a previous therapist, I realized there was a common theme: the therapist wasn't listening to what they wanted. If they tell you they've been having calf pain and you lightly and briefly go over the gastrocnemious, you are ignoring their request for more attention to that area. Remember their stated pain areas, check in at least once on your pressure, and give the massage that they want.

3. Ending

I usually ended massage face up with

- neck work

- a gentle scalp massage

- face massage

- a few moments of breathing while softly holding their temples

Then I said thank you.

## Closing Up Your Time Together

Most spas have client in a robe to go from the relaxation lounge to your room. If so, as they are relaxing with eyes shut, place the robe across their body and slippers or shoes beside the table, assuming they are face up. If they are face down at end, put robe on a nearby chair that they can grab when they sit up. You don't want them to get up to a cool room when they are relaxed and have to walk around in a dimly lit, unfamiliar room, trying to recall where they put their shoes. The longer they can keep this feeling of relaxation, the better.

If they came in wearing their street clothes, leave their clothing where it was placed. No one wants to have their underwear fall out of his or her pile of clothes. Or, there may be jewelry in a pocket that could fall out. Raise the lights slightly so they can see where their clothing is.

It is best to gently touch the top or their head or hand and let them know that you will be outside the door waiting for them. As you hopefully have another client waiting, you don't want them to fall back to sleep or remain on the bed meditating for a half an hour. As wonderful as it is to help someone relax, the spa is a business and they like to keep busy. Often you have ten minutes between clients, so the timing of this between-time needs to feel relaxed, yet be quick and efficient.

## On Time Ending

Ending on time is huge in a spa for several reasons. The client may have to be somewhere and be expecting to leave at the preset time. They don't have a watch on so are depending on you. They may have another appointment at the spa, which they want to be on time for and you don't want to mess up a co-worker's schedule. And even if you think that you have no massage after this, and it is okay to end late, you could have been booked with something while in massage. Finally, if you give extra time, the client may expect this next time. Or they may have a friend who was receiving a service at the same time. If your client comes out later from a longer massage, the friend will feel cheated and probably complain. So, end on time.

When the client comes out of the room, either be ready with a glass of water, or be leading them to the lounge and offer it there. Drinking water after a massage is crucial. Doing so can avoid having an achy body from the release of toxins, as you most likely learned in school. Let the client know this by telling them to drink extra water that day to avoid being sore.

<u>You Did It!</u>

Another congratulations here! You have just given an awesome massage, helped someone to relax, and relieved some of his or her pain and stress. What wonderful things to be able to do for another human being. Before they leave, make the attempt to have them come back for another beneficial treatment. The next chapter will help you learn how.

# How Do You Get Your Client To Rebook
## Chapter Nine

You've just given someone a massage and they feel great. They are relaxed, peaceful, and free of all that stress they came in with. Wow. All of that in just one hour. Wouldn't you want to come back for more?

1. Health Benefits

As you lead them back to the Relaxation Lounge, continue the spa experience by keeping your voice quiet. Ask if they feel good. Now is a good time to gently let them know that you suggest they come back for whatever they need and when. As they are in a relaxed state of mind, and you are the one who helped to get them there, they will be open to doing what you tell them. This is not about mind control; it is a time that they are open to truly taking in the health benefits of massage. Here is a partial list of massage benefits:

- relieves stress

- releases body pain

- reduces blood pressure and heart rate

- increases lymph flow

- reduces edema

- relieves and reduces some kinds of back pain

- reduces anxiety

You know how beneficial massage is for the body; that's why you became a massage therapist. Pass on the wonderful news that the bliss your client is feeling goes beyond simply feeling good, it is also good for them.

Let the client know that they should continue in caring for themselves.  To ensure the health of a body, just like a car, pet, or plants, it needs regular maintenance. The acceptance of massage as a requirement to healthy living has become more accepted in our society.  However, many people still view massage as a luxury to partake in once a year, while on vacation.  Let your client know the health benefits of a monthly massage.

2. How Often To Come In

My guidelines were: if there is extensive pain, tight muscles, or stress that really needs attention, the client needs to schedule an appointment for next week. If they are in need of normal maintenance, then a monthly massage may be perfect.

Let them know that rebooking now will keep them on the path of a healthy body. If they wait to rebook they will probably forget. Now is the time to do it.

Many people are unable to schedule a month in advance due to a changing schedule. If this is the case, say something like, "this is October, so be sure to call back to reschedule in November." Naming the months makes it more real and a part of their routine.

Don't be pushy here but know that what you have to offer is crucial to their health. Believe and know that you are offering a benefit that will help them in their life.

3. Ensure Comfort

When you drop them off in the relaxation room, do what you can to ensure their comfort before you leave. Bring water, an extra pillow or blanket, a magazine. Ask if there is anything else you can do for them before you leave. These little touches take just a minute of your time, and can make a big difference in having them come back to you for their massage. We all want to be pampered, loved and cared for. Let them know that they are worth your time.

The extra touches given toward their comfort will also translate to bigger tips for you. Again, we are here to help people, but can only do this if our bills are paid — we need to make a good living at massage so that we can stay healthy and remain in the business.

Offer your card. Let them know that you will notify the spa receptionist when they should re-book so they won't have to worry about it. Speak gently, not pushing anything on them. What you are offering them is about their health and well-being. You are giving a gift and expecting them to take it, with out being pushy.

Say good-bye, use their name, and give a nice handshake or hug if appropriate. Tell them thank you for coming in and that you look forward to seeing them again.

Race To The Front

Depending on whether or not you have a client, and how much time you have will obviously effect what you can do now.  You may have to race, but in the long run the extra effort will be worth it.  Find a way to get to the spa receptionist to tell him or her when you want the client to rebook. If a particular lotion was used, especially if you discussed the product with the client, you can leave it with the receptionist for her or him to sale.

If you happen to be at the front desk when your client comes out, let the client know that the receptionist is ready to book their next appointment. Speak as though you expect that this will happen. Show your clients the products that you are recommending that they take home that day.

Then say goodbye and leave. Let the receptionist continue with their job. If you are standing behind the counter as they check out, the client may feel like you are pushing them into buying the suggested product and waiting to be sure they rebook with you. Also, it is awkward if you are hanging around when the receptionist asks if they would like to leave a tip and how much.

Spa receptionists usually get a small commission in booking and sales. It is to their benefit if a client comes back, and when they buy something. Hopefully, you will have a great receptionist who will continue your work and get you a re-booking.

Now get back to your room and have it cleaned and ready for your next client. You are on a massage roll!

Leaving a Job

Chapter Ten

When you leave a spa job, never burn bridges.
In the more expensive day spas, it is a very tight,
small community. The last spa I worked at, after
being in the business for several years, I discovered
that I had previously worked with every therapist
there. Had I had problems with just one co-worker, I
might not have been hired.

If you have decided to leave the spa industry to start your own practice, ask your supervisor if you can tell your spa regulars where you are going. Some places are open to this practice. But if the spa tell you no, respect their wishes. You want to be able to go back there if your new place doesn't work out, or if you need extra money and want to return on a part-time basis. The best outcome is to be on good terms with every spa you've worked at.

It is a good idea when you leave to ask if you can remain on-call. Who knows if you may want to return because the new situation didn't work out. Also, spas often book a party and need extra therapists for a day. Or someone will call in sick at the last moment. If you are available, you may have just found a way to make some extra money.

## Wonders Of The Industry

The massage industry is a wonderful opportunity to make an income while serving people. Having worked with chiropractors, physical therapists, and on my own, the luxury spa is by far the easiest most lucrative option. The settings are calm, beautiful, and peaceful. The clients were primarily there to relax and you get to be a part of their tranquil day. With the base pay, commission and tips, I made a good living.

I hope this book has been beneficial and will land you a terrific job that you will be happy in. I wish you the best of luck in your massage therapist career. Thank you for reading this book.

Please go to Amazon.com and leave an honest review.

The best advice I can give you I heard from one of the best therapists I ever had the pleasure to work with, "Love your client".

Namaste